The Secrets of Modern Acupuncture

How to maximize your health and wellbeing

Dr. Justin Newman, CPC, MS, OMD

www.theBanyanHolistic.com

OVERVIEW

Forward, by Dr. Daniel Medvedov, MS, OMD, PhD
Introduction

Concluding Thoughts and Brief Biography

Forward,
Dr. Daniel Medvedov, MS, OMD, PhD

After years of being a friend and colleague of Dr. Justin Newman, and working together in our daily labors, I realized that the Good Doctor lives simultaneously in three realms: a spiritual one, a scientific one, and a poetic one. When asked to say some words on his attainments, a brief account would be the following, "This is truly a Doctor!"

The scientific view allows us to have access to the most intricate and complex matters, and to solve complicated problems if blessed with wit and a capacity for synthesis. At the same time, the modesty of a person with vast knowledge shows that some subject matters are, and remain, possibly beyond our ken. I have such a feeling when I think and contemplate the medical labors of Dr. Justin Newman.

The capacity to describe in a few words a complex subject matter is the testimony of deep understanding of the value, principles, and full extent of that subject. To transmit it to the public in clear terms and precise description is yet another tenet – few are endowed with that capacity for synthesis and an analytical approach. This book, *The Secrets of Modern Acupuncture*, has a scent of the breeze coming from a sea of knowledge. Indeed, it is more difficult to write a synopsis of a complex subject than to write a book of 1,000 pages!

Introduction

There is a great deal of speculation as to the true origins of acupuncture. Whether the art and science of acupuncture is an ancient medical system or is a considerably more recent invention is of little consequence. It has become one of the most widely administered, natural, and holistic traditional systems in existence.

Acupuncture works by stimulating specific zones on the body with hair-thin needles, in order to provoke the body's own healing capabilities. In this way, acupuncture therapy can assist the skilled physician whenever he or she is treating medical issues. These treatable medical issues number in the hundreds, according to the World Health Organization and the National Institutes of Health.

I have been involved with the field of holistic healthcare since 1992, and have always maintained a holistic perspective. In my professional experience, as a licensed doctor of oriental medicine and holistic primary healthcare provider, there has recently been an incredible rise in openness and motivation from people in the mainstream. Familiarity with acupuncture is now commonplace, significantly more so than when I began practicing medicine. Since then, there has been an exponential rise in the number of people that are discovering how acupuncture can help them to live pain free, more relaxed, comfortable, energetic lives, and enable them to reach a higher level of overall health and wellbeing.

Out of several, perhaps the most popular system of acupuncture is featured within traditional Chinese medicine (TCM), one of few remaining traditional medical systems. Even within TCM, there are a vast number of individual lineages: scholar and physician driven; family and local schools of thought; and, several microsystems such as auricular acupuncture (all points are on the ear). There are also some subsystems that still retain much of the shamanic, animist precursors to TCM. There is similar profundity within the Ayurvedic medical system of India, given its connection to the Himalayan system of Bönpo. Another example would be the Olmec-Mayan traditional medical system. Each of the aforementioned systems includes acupuncture.

Acupuncture therapy has undergone extensive research as well as widespread practice and development. There are now many specializations of modern medicine to which acupuncture is being applied. Electrical stimulation with acupuncture and laserpuncture are among the newer innovations. Additionally, acupuncture anesthesia for surgical procedures has become a well-established niche. Currently, the medical paradigm is shifting toward one of Integrative Medicine. This is more beneficial for all of us, now that collaboration between the mainstream and the holistic is occurring. However, at the end of the day, we might reflect on the physician's oath, "First, do no harm."

01

A comprehensive medical system

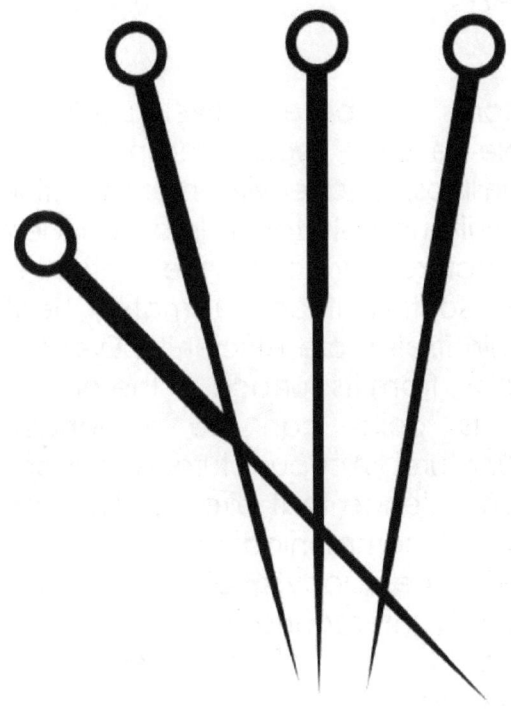

Acupuncture is used to effectively treat a large number of health concerns. The efficacy of acupoint therapy has been demonstrated repeatedly, regardless of the type of ailment or level of severity. As a perfect complement, acupuncture has also been shown to work well when combined with other therapies, such as massage therapy.

Symptoms can be effectively addressed on multiple levels – body, feelings, thoughts, relationships, and environmental influences are simultaneously taken into consideration. Acupuncture leverages the patient's own system, so that it can ultimately heal and maintain itself more efficiently. Every part of the body, from its surface to the organs and even its cells, can be influenced by acupuncture. Acupuncture is a complete medical science that directly stimulates the intricate communication system that supports the body's other systems. This network is interconnected throughout the entire body, and affects every aspect of who we are.

Acupuncture is comprehensive. Therapy can have profound effects on the overall functioning of each patient. However, therapy addresses more than only the presenting symptoms, it also focuses on the root causes of a patient's medical concerns. Furthermore, it would be desirable to prevent diseases from manifesting in the first place. An old adage states, **"If the person's system is functioning in harmony, there will be no sickness, aging, or death."** This suggests that a patient should not wait until their symptoms become more chronic and debilitating to seek proper medical care and support.

02

Comfortable holistic methods and applications

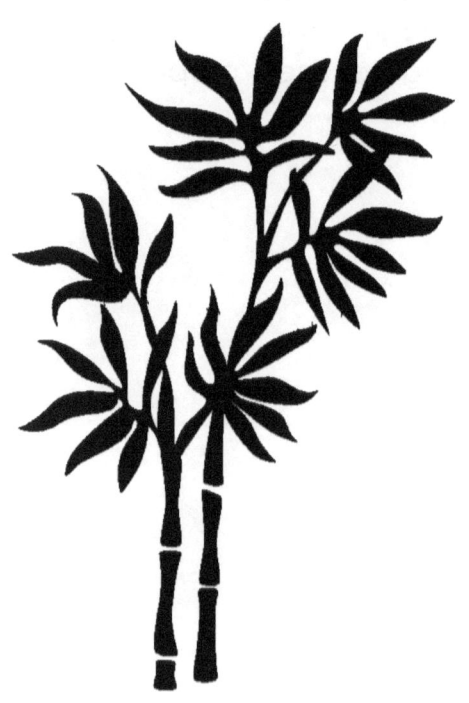

Acupuncture is holistic in both its philosophical and therapeutic frameworks. **Holistic means, "whole person."** As such, acupuncture takes into account every aspect of each individual patient. This is crucial since we are not simply a body, but a complex, multifaceted, functioning entity. Even when simply considering an individual's body, we also take into account consciousness, beliefs and social paradigms, even the impact of countless operations that occur on an atomic or quantum level.

An insightful acupuncture physician might choose from a number of diagnostic tools to find the pattern within the presenting symptoms. The acupuncturist will seek to determine the root cause or causes and the origins of the symptom pattern. The physician will then seek a path toward pattern resolution, and simultaneously nurture the ability of patients to regain and strengthen their constitution. Acupuncture that is performed in a healthcare center should have an atmosphere that is conducive to relaxation. This type of experience can optimize both overall comfort level as well as any therapeutic benefits from their visit. Under these soothing conditions, it is common for most clients to actually fall asleep and rest deeply during their experiences with acupuncture.

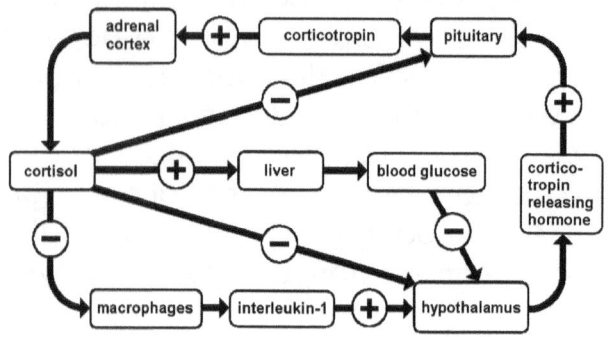

Biochemistry of the Metabolic Process
J.A. Illingworth, University of Leeds

03

Origins of Integrative Medicine

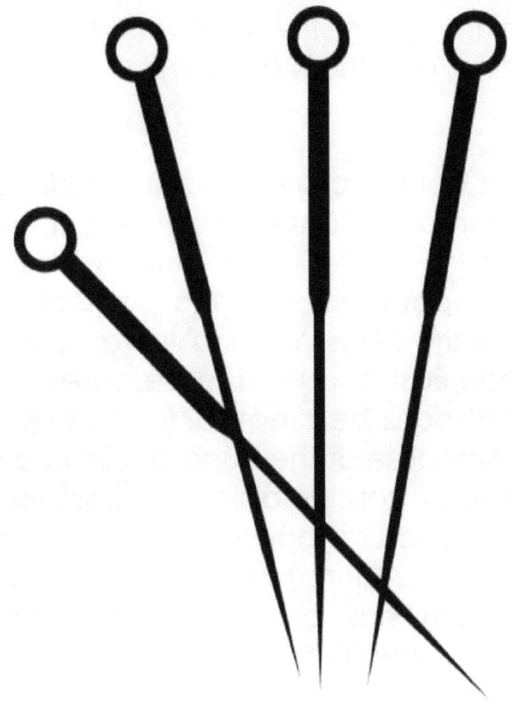

The current trend in the practice of modern medicine is that we integrate the mainstream with the holistic. This paradigm is referred to as Integrative Medicine. The Consortium of Academic Health Centers for Integrative Medicine was founded in 1999, and by 2015 included 60 members, such as Johns Hopkins University School of Medicine, Duke University School of Medicine, Georgetown University School of Medicine, and the Mayo Clinic.

Modern acupuncture was first introduced to European physicians and scholars in the 17th century. However, not until widespread interest appeared, with the political events of the early 1970s allowing travel restrictions between East and West to be eased, would a springboard be created. In the past thirty years, because of the huge public interest in this subject, considerable scientific research on acupuncture has been carried out - although much remains to be done. This momentum has paved the way for the integrative healthcare model that is finally emerging.

It is commonplace to see acupuncture physicians, and other holistic professionals, in clinics, hospitals, and medical schools, working alongside allopathic physicians. Medical programs typically direct students into familiarization and training in the use of specific complementary methods, such as acupuncture. The National Center for Complementary and Integrative Health continues to nurture this approach to resolving disease and maintaining health.

04

Proven, time-tested results

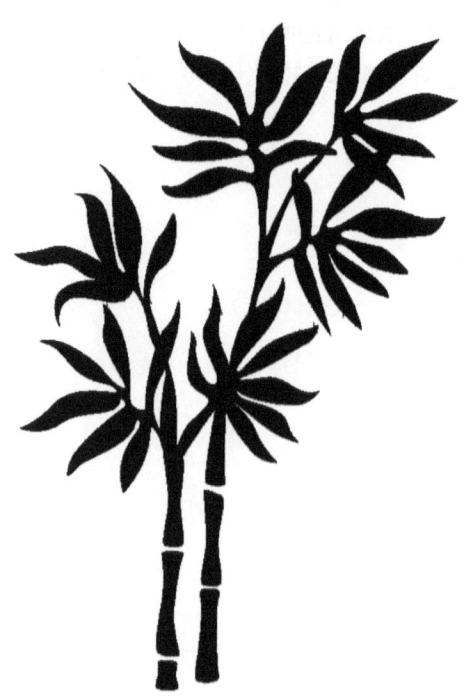

Throughout the years, there have been innumerable studies, which can attest to the efficacy of acupuncture. Treatments on a wide array of health concerns have been examined. There is both an extensive empirical record as well as anecdotal evidence, across a multigenerational lineage of physicians and scholars. Published and peer-reviewed documentation support and reinforce the assertion that acupuncture is a proven, effective medical procedure.

In recent years, both the **World Health Organization (WHO)** and the **National Institutes of Health (NIH)** have released independent assessments, which concluded that acupuncture is helpful in treating hundreds of medical issues. Furthermore, many randomized, controlled clinical trials, along with meta-analyses of the effectiveness of acupuncture in the treatment of various diseases have been conducted. There is now a much higher level of corroborating evidence. This has all occurred in the 15 years following the publication of the WHO report.

Acupuncture has become widely accepted into the mainstream. Consequently, a paradigm shift is occurring: the current healthcare model is being defined as **Integrative Medicine,** which is when the conventional and holistic systems work together. Currently, medical programs throughout the world feature both academic and clinical training in how to make the best use of this integrated approach. For those who find it hard to believe, it is important to note that acupuncture has been used in pediatric medicine, veterinary medicine, and with unconscious patients. This strongly suggests that there is little likelihood of any placebo effect from acupuncture.

05

Convenient for any lifestyle

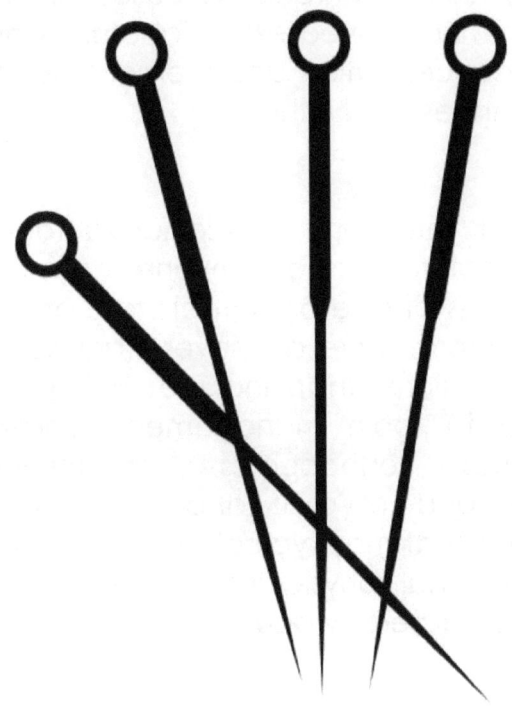

Acupuncture complements multiple goals - If you have an injury, acupuncture reduces pain, inflammation, and promotes repair. If you have panic and anxiety or other strong emotional patterns, acupuncture reduces the effects of stress on your body, while facilitating a calmer, clearer mind. Acupuncture is also effective when treating fertility issues, chronic diseases (including autoimmune diseases), diabetes, cancer, poor concentration and memory, hormonal imbalances, and lethargy.

One of the considerable advantages of acupuncture is that anyone can use it, regardless of age or current state of health. Furthermore, there are several acupuncture specializations that include but are not limited to: pain management; pediatrics; geriatrics; orthopedics; endocrinology; fertility and ob-gyn; and oncology. The ailments that may typically be addressed by conventional physicians or therapists can also be treated by acupuncture.

Using acupuncture can facilitate other aspects of a person's life. Depending on the desired goals, acupuncture can improve focus, clarity, and self-motivation. It also boosts overall energy levels. This results in greater balance, connectedness, and an enhanced ability to flow with the various challenges that will be faced throughout the day. Acupuncture can lead to peak performance. Our goals can be more easily and swiftly achieved by incorporating acupuncture as part of a lifestyle regimen.

06

Simultaneously working on mind and body

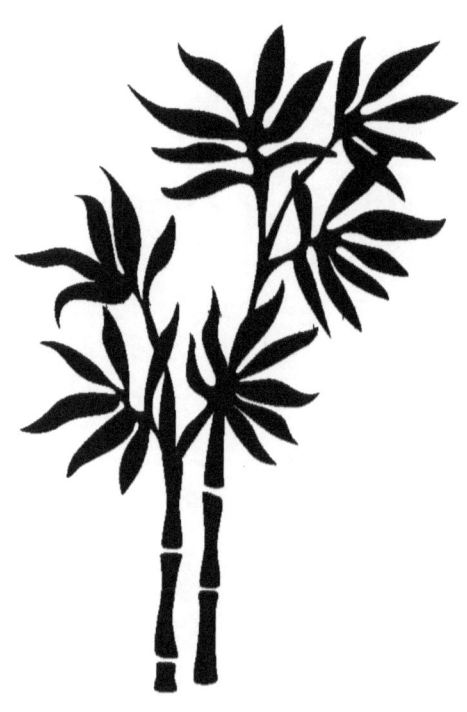

Acupuncture has measureable effects on both the mind and the body. The interconnected, harmonious functioning of these two aspects of a person is vitally important when assessing their level of wellness and wellbeing. After all, the mind will perceive stimuli and then relay information to the body, so that the individual can respond in healthy, productive, appropriate ways. From these interactions, the emotions are produced, which in turn affect the quality of a person's life and relationships.

When the microscopic point of an acupuncture needle is introduced to the body, there are quite a few immediate changes that take place. First, the circulation, muscle tone, and electrical conductivity of the area are affected. Second, the nervous system is stimulated to respond – this incorporates the corresponding neurotransmitters and numerous endocrine hormones involved. Third, the immune system is activated by the invasion of a needle, which leads to an increase in white blood cell production. And finally, the brain is triggered to release endorphins. **Enhanced relaxation and a sense of inner balance and calm are**

typically experienced when receiving acupuncture.

These are common occurrences for the acupuncture patient. As the body adapts to the changes that are therapeutically provoked, we find that the organ systems start to work closer toward their optimum. The stimulated organ(s) and other systems of the body will tend to integrate more effectively with each other. At this point, a person may find it easier to sustain a more refined and functional level of wellness and wellbeing.

07

The simple and direct approach

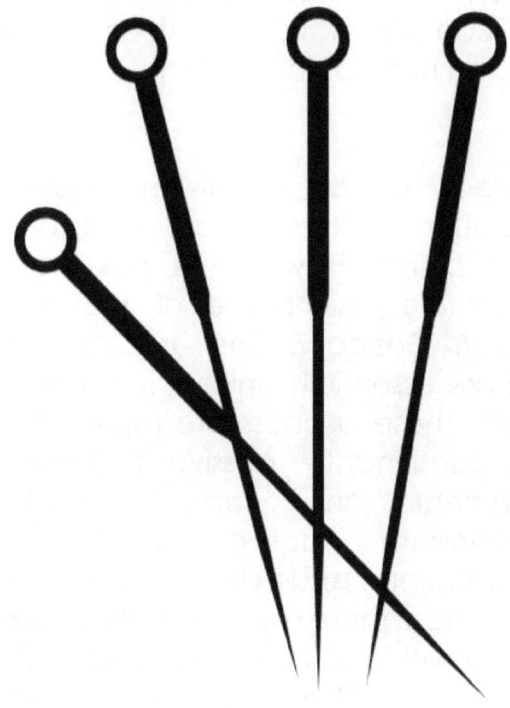

While acupuncture may appear to be incredibly sophisticated, intricate, and elegant, it is actually very simple and direct in its approach. The acupuncturist merely has to find and manipulate the appropriate point or points on the body. Due to the interconnected network between the body and mind, we often find examples when less is more. For instance, just one acupuncture point can dramatically affect the entire body and mind of the patient.

The great masters of this medical system would often perform therapy using only one or two points. How is this possible? With acupuncture, the name of the game is harmony. Basically, the body's systems, which are essentially unified, have two main aspects. These aspects are represented by the predominantly passive functions, like nourishment and support, and the predominantly active functions, like transformation and development. Yin & Yang. When these two aspects operate in harmony with each other, a person will have health and wellbeing; if not, disease and malcontent.

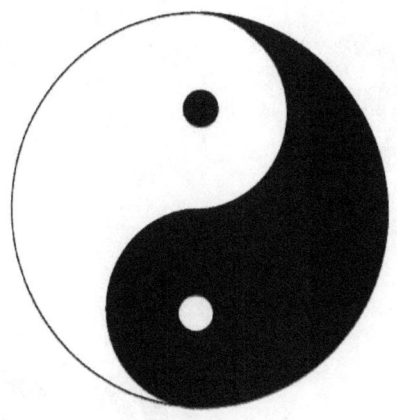

A single acupuncture point can restore harmony.

08

Transform. Harmonize.

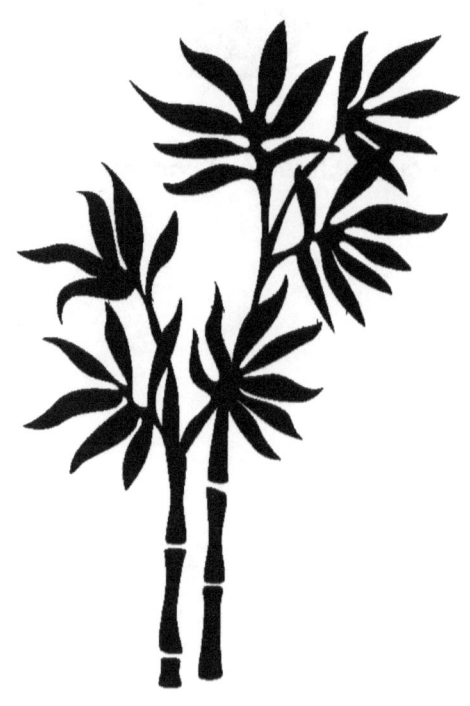

An outstanding characteristic about acupuncture therapy is that it is a medical system that encourages the proper functioning of the body's own anatomy and physiology. It assists with what the body *wants* to be doing, whenever it is free from any internal or external saboteurs. In this way, the body can be restored to an improved level of functioning, and be better able to maintain itself.

Acupuncture helps the body to find its proper balance point. Balance is required for ideal functioning. This is called homeostasis. When all processes are in balance and harmony the body functions at its best. It becomes progressively easier to navigate daily challenges as well as those that occur throughout our lives.

Finally, acupuncture is used to regulate the functioning of the body, so that any excesses or deficiencies that may appear can be safely and quickly resolved. This is important because there are many factors that can affect our health, whenever the system becomes compromised. Injury and trauma, chronic illness, poorly managed stress, exposure to toxins, and influences from our immediate environment are some examples of what might be compromising factors. Acupuncture optimizes performance and restores the body to a higher level of wellness.

"Homeostatic reactions are inevitable and automatic if the system is functioning properly... and maintained by many systems operating together."

– Emeritus Professor Kelvin Rodolfo, University of Illinois

09

Rejuvenation

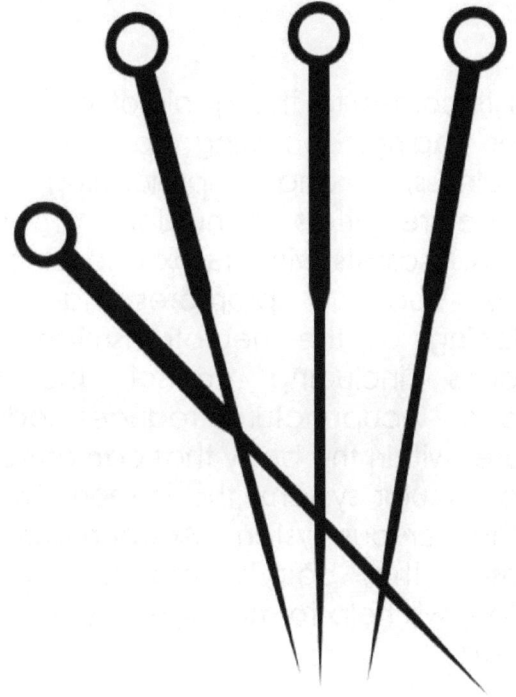

There is perhaps nothing more extraordinary than acupuncture's ability to counteract the effects of aging in the body. As previously mentioned, the ideal and optimal functioning of the body can become compromised if not correctly managed. Acupuncture resolves the impact that various traumas and influences can have on the individual's system over time.

When it comes to the goals of combating cellular aging, boosting longevity and youthfulness, and prolonging life, acupuncture offers a number of helpful solutions. It assists with detox and cleansing of the body. It promotes harmonious functioning of the neurotransmitters and hormones, including cortisol, the stress hormone. Acupuncture reduces adverse pressures within the body that can affect the cardiovascular system, the immune system, and the nervous system. Acupuncture also regulates the body's metabolism and therefore will help to manage any demands for energy.

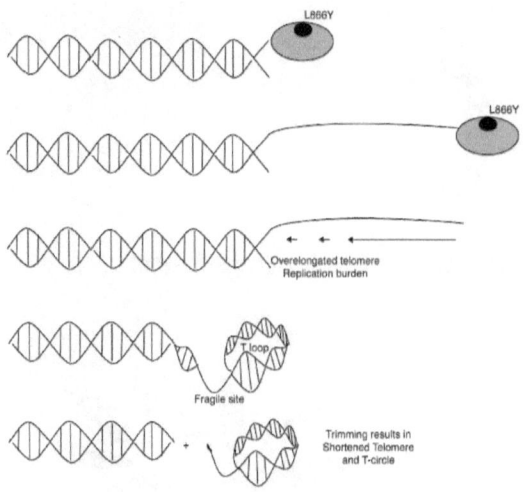

[**Regulation of telomere length and homeostasis by telomerase enzyme processivity.**

Yasmin D'Souza, Catherine Lauzon, Tsz Wai Chu, Chantal Autexier.
J Cell Sci 2013 126: 676-687; doi: 10.1242/jcs.119297.]

10

Natural, no adverse side effects

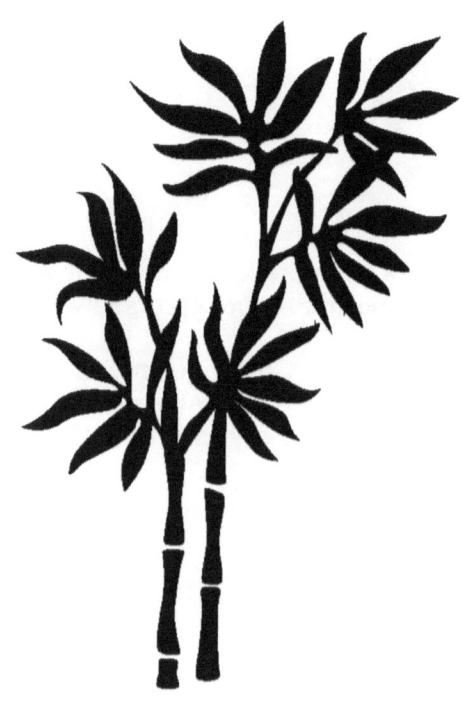

Acupuncture is a medical system that provides a way to resolve health concerns and symptoms, without the need for pharmaceutical intervention. This is not to necessarily advocate that patients immediately stop taking their prescription medications. Pharmaceuticals can be useful for emergency or acute issues. However, an ultimate goal for health providers should be to ultimately use no medications, *rather than continually adding more.*

The body's natural ability to regulate and heal itself is assisted by acupuncture. This is a superior choice for the long-term promotion of health and wellbeing. It complements the ways in which the body *prefers to be functioning,* when at its optimal level of wellness. The perfect design of the body allows for the clearing of symptoms and maintaining a good quality of life.

With acupuncture, there are two main side effects, both of which are positive:
- Acupuncture boosts the immune system and stimulates the body to produce more white blood cells. This helps to fight off infections, eliminate toxins and damaged cells, and even

reduces the proliferation of cancerous cells.

- Acupuncture triggers the brain to release endorphins, which are neurotransmitters that help to manage pain and stress.

With these benefits, and many others, acupuncture helps a patient to function with a calmer, clearer, and more relaxed state of being. Navigating the sea of life becomes a more harmonious endeavor....

Concluding Thoughts

There are many avenues you can explore when faced with a medical or other kind of personal challenge. Be empowered to make the choice that best suits you, your lifestyle, and your ultimate goals. Navigating the vast number of possibilities, while sorting through the mountain of detailed information that continually surrounds us, requires expert guidance. There is perhaps nowhere more explicit in this regard than when facing medical decisions.

For investing your time and effort into this work, I would personally like to invite you to contact me for scheduling an introductory priced acupuncture session whenever in our area, to subscribe to our webinar, blog, and podcasting channels, and to otherwise gain more information about holistic medicine -

Wellness@theBanyanHolistic.com

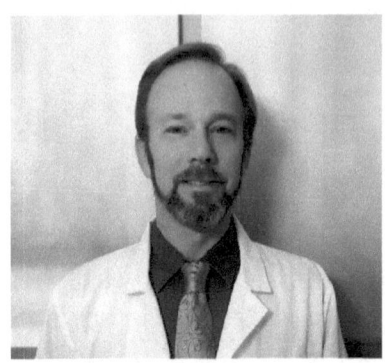

Dr. Justin Newman, CPC, MS, OMD

Dr. Newman is a triple major, pre-med graduate of the University of Miami, and has been a licensed physician specializing in traditional Chinese medicine, acupuncture, and holistic healthcare for over 16 years.

With 23 years of experience in the field of holistic primary healthcare, Dr. Newman continues to strive in further enriching the community, while implementing programs that guide clients into simultaneous empowerment and fulfillment within their lives. The unique framework of his approach promotes health and harmony on every level – physical, emotional, mental, social, and spiritual. He presents a modernized, reimagined innovation based on time tested and proven healthcare systems.

Dr. Newman has cultivated relationships with professionals in many fields, so that this vision can be truly integrated with the mainstream. Having established university-level teaching experience, Dr. Newman has had numerous invitations to share his expertise on radio and television, for various institutions such as the United Way, the Miami-Dade County School Board, and many non-profit and government agencies as well. He is also a quoted authority on the subject of Chinese medicine and holistic healthcare. Many have found that his simple and convenient methods naturally encourage cooperation and productivity. To complement his medical and research practice, Dr. Newman conducts regular classes in aikido, yoga and meditation, and immortality philosophy.